10

Minute Yogi

The World's Most Efficient Yoga Manual

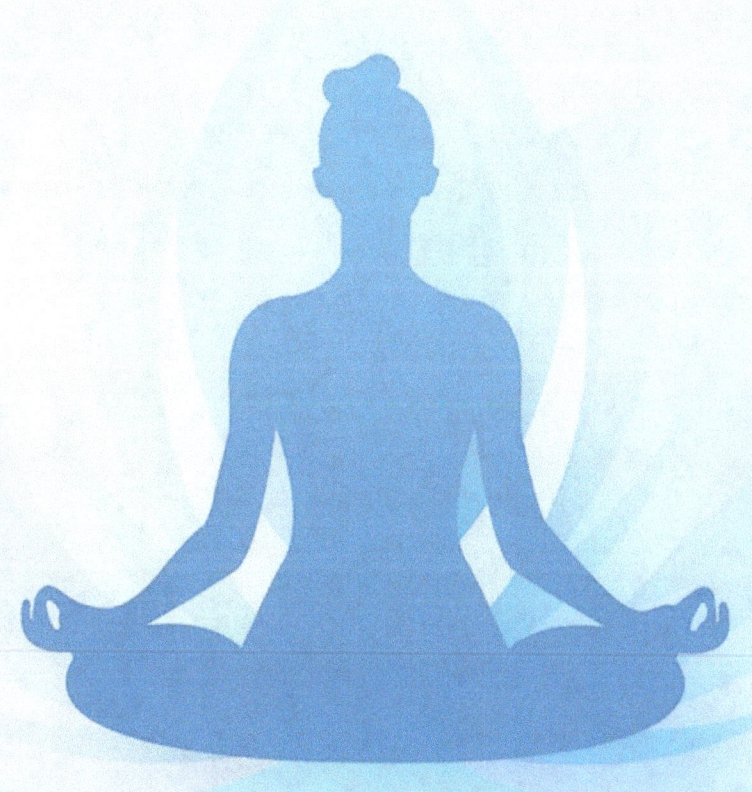

TRENT ANTHONY
(HARDCORE YOGI)

10 Minute Yogi

The World's Most Efficient Yoga Manual

TRENT ANTHONY

(HARDCORE YOGI)

BLURB

This is the most efficient yoga manual to date. Slick, to the point, yet somehow encapsulating the breadth of this tradition. In just 40 pages, Trent covers five main areas:

Defining Yoga and the Eight Limbs – Physical postures are but one limb. Learn the ancient foundation laid out by the Sages.

Asana (posture) – Trent shares some deep principles for building the perfect posture, split into two categories: anatomical techniques and psychedelic techniques. In the appendix, he provides a list of foundational asanas, including images and step-by-step instructions.

Pranayama (breathwork) – Learn the mechanisms of healthy breathing, and how, counterintuitively, breathing less is a sign of superior health. He then provides exercises that will help you navigate the wide world of pranayama.

Meditation – Trent starts by grappling with the slippery definition of meditation. Thankfully, he pins that sucker down. We then look at the benefits of meditation through the lens of a western scientist and an eastern mystic. At the end is a list of techniques that are simple yet effective at centering the Self.

The Yogi's Guide to Lifelong Practice – There are many puzzle pieces that will help you fit yoga into your daily life. Consistency, group practice, independent practice, and adequate theoretical knowledge are all factors that will ensure your life-long commitment. Here's a goal: Do yoga every day until your last. This section will help you with such a goal.

From the big picture to step-by-step, Trent unpacks the fundamentals in a way that is fun, fresh, and original. This is the perfect crash course for a busy person who wants to achieve optimal well-being.

ABOUT THE AUTHOR

———— ⚜ ————

Trent is a dedicated polymath and internationally accredited yoga teacher. He is most specialized in yoga and hip-hop music, yet has a broad love of movement, music, writing, and speaking. These outlets touch on the themes of health and fitness, personal development, the spiritual path, and sustainable living. You can find his works on www.hardcoreyogi.com.

TABLE OF CONTENTS

INTRODUCTION

This book went from 90,000 words to 10,000 words. Far beyond yoga, I voyaged across many domains—from Ayurveda to nutrition and fitness, to mysticism and psychology, and ended the tour with social sustainability. The topics flowed out of me, and I believe the ideas are still valid. So, why did I hack away at my precious? The seed was planted by writing educator, William Zinsser, when he said that a piece of writing cannot cover everything. It cannot even cover a whole topic, let alone multiple topics. Therefore, it pays to know what slice of the topic you intend to write about, and to do it very well. Since yoga is my specialisation, I kept the first few chapters which laid down the foundations of yoga. I then chiseled away at those chapters.

I believe every great work is a synthesis. My favourite books are little more than 200 pages, sometimes even less. I call these books my "bibles". Such books are concise and profound—a high economy of meaning. Maximum signal, minimal noise. I hope this book hits such a note.

What does yoga mean to me? I'm not talking about a definition. Rather, what role does it play in my life? For some, it is a form of physical conditioning. It has been for me, but it's more than that. For some, it is a physical therapy, assisting with functional movement and pain relief. Again, it has been for me, but it's more than that. It can be a way to de-stress and relax. It can be a way to prime the system for meditation and spiritual gains. For me, it is all these things and more. Yoga is a form of nourishment, a staple in the good life. It is a technology and an art form, which serves one major purpose—to optimize the human being. There are many ways to optimize your life, but to me, yoga is the most foundational and holistic. This is not a sales pitch. It is my truth told raw. Yoga is a leverage point that makes everything else flow into place.

CHAPTER 1 – WHAT IS YOGA?

Defining Yoga

Yoga comes from the Sanskrit word 'yog', which means to yolk, bind, or unite. In his famous book, *Light on Yoga*, BKS Iyenga says that yoga is the unification of our physical, mental, and emotional faculties, with our personal will and the will of God. In other words, every element of us moves in one direction, aligned with the interest of ourselves and the All. This is achieved through purification of the body, mind, and spirit.

The Eight Limbs

First described in *The Yoga Sutras of Patanjali*, "The eight limbs of yoga" is the essential blueprint of the yogic system. It is a set of practices relating to lifestyle, physical movement, breath, and meditation, gearing us toward our highest spiritual potential.

1. Yamas: Ethical Disciplines
- Ahimsa (non-harming)
- Satya (truthfulness)
- Asteya (non-stealing)
- Aparigraha (non-possessiveness, detachment)
- Brahmacharya (moderation)

2. Niyamas: Self Disciplines
- Tapas (fiery ambition to be our best)
- Santosha (contentment)
- Saucha (cleanliness)
- Svadhyaya (self-study)
- Ishvara Pranidhana (study/reflection of the divine)

3: Asana: Posture

4: Pranayama: Breath

5: Pratyahara: Turning the senses within

6: Dharana: Concentration on a single point

7: Dhyana: Meditation, sustained concentration on a single point

8: Samadhi: Absorption in one's meditation. Pure presence, consciousness, and love. The self and the environment become one. Mystical states may ensue

Let us encapsulate the eight limbs of yoga in a paragraph rather than bullet points. Imagine the yogi has been living an ethical life, staying active, clean, disciplined, and well-studied. He then takes his seat for meditation. His posture is cross-legged with his spine erect, balanced, and comfortable. The energy is flowing freely. He closes his eyes and notices his breath, which is slow, deep, and energising. It fills his pelvis and lifts his spine, raising energy up through the head and beyond. His senses are turned within as he maintains focus on the movement of breath and body. In this vacuum of focus, he introduces a mantra: Sat Nam – Truth is My Name. Repeating the mantra, he becomes so absorbed in the meditation that his personal problems disappear. He vanishes and becomes one with the object of meditation. In this case, Sat Nam. Later, he emerges with a deep inhale and opening of the eyes. His energy is blissful, serene, awake. His perception is so pure that he can sense the miracle of existence all around him. Such is the essence of yoga.

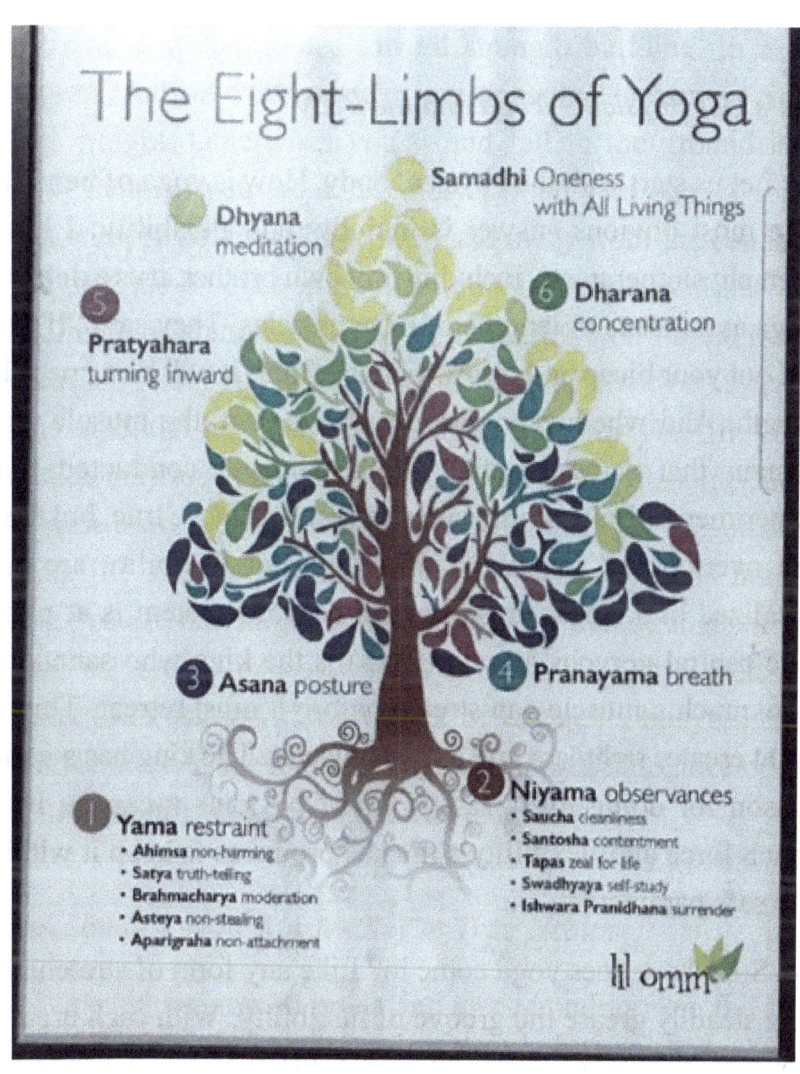

Beyond the human being, prana gives life to the birds and the bees, the trees and the mountains. It is the substrate of all reality.

In humans, qi and prana is the force that flows through our bodies. This system of energy is referred to as the "energy body", "subtle body", or "pranic body". In western terms, it includes many functions such as kinetic energy, thermal energy, electricity, blood, ATP, glucose, hormones, neurotransmitters, nerve impulses, and respiration. Western culture has many fine-grain models to describe what happens in the body, whereas qi describes the unified system of these parts. Because, in truth, the different western models affect one another. For instance, your neurotransmitters affect your hormones, and your hormones affect your glucose metabolism. These systems rise and fall together, feeding off each other's harmony or disharmony.

The goal of yoga and qigong is to work directly on the pranic body. By restoring a functional, harmonious flow in the pranic body, in turn, we restore harmony to every bodily system. It is like a master key.

Have you ever noticed that an undesirable state often manifests as a "kink" in your energy body? Perhaps it's a feeling of tension, dullness, or excitation, which interrupts the smooth flow of your circuitry. Introduce yoga. When you consciously move and breathe with grace, you are mobilizing prana, i.e. blood, oxygen, hormones, etc. You are resetting your entire system, returning to a peaceful equilibrium. You have removed the blockage that was troubling you. The dust settles, and everything returns to its proper place. Here you find a state of happiness, for happiness is the absence of dysfunction.

Chapter 2 – Asana (Posture)

From The Ground Up: Asana Families

When approaching the big wide world of yoga asanas, it is useful to know about asana families. Each asana family is like a food group, varying in their structure, function, and benefit. Thankfully, none of them contain empty calories. Below is a list of the asana families. In each yoga session, we generally perform them in this order:

- Warm-up flows and salutations
- Standing postures
- Backbends
- Abdominal and core (can be omitted)
- Arm balances (can be omitted)
- Forward folds and hip openers
- Twists
- Inversions

It is useful to know the asana families because they provide a map for starting your practice. You can begin with the easiest and most foundational postures within each asana family. As you begin to master and understand the foundational postures, you can progress to more challenging postures within that family.

Another advantage of understanding asana families is that they each benefit different muscle groups, organs, and bodily functions. This allows you to pick and choose a practice suited to your needs for the day, or to create a well-rounded practice. Generally, salutations and standing postures warm up the body. Backbends and arm balances are stimulating and invigorating. Forward folds and hip openers are calming and relaxing. Twists aid with digestive fire. Over time, you will feel the way that different postures affect your energy. You can then intuitively blend postures based on your needs and desires at that time.

Constructing The Asana: Anatomical Techniques and Psychedelic Techniques

This section contains concepts and techniques that will serve you in mastering each asana. These ideas can be applied to any asana under the sun. In fact, they can probably be applied to any form of movement. I have split them into two broad categories—anatomical techniques and psychedelic techniques. When I say psychedelic techniques, I am referring to the more feminine, intuitive, holistic approaches to yoga practice. On the other hand, anatomical techniques provide a grounded logical basis for constructing the asana.

Anatomical Techniques

Aligning From the Ground Up

When entering the posture and refining it, consider the placement of several major joints in the body. The feet, ankles, knees, hips, spine, chest and shoulders, arms, neck, and head should all come into account. The aim is to have each of these body parts in the correct position for that posture. Each posture has different alignment cues. For example, in triangle pose (trikonasana), you want to have the chest and shoulder aligned directly above your knee. In tadasana, mountain pose, you want your head and neck directly above your spine. Learn the alignment cues by listening to your instructor and personally studying each posture. This book can contribute to such a study.

Aligning in 3D

In the first principle, "aligning from the ground up", I described the essential body parts to focus on. These included all the major joints from head to toe. I then suggested that we align these joints from "the ground up", which is the vertical axis. But in our 3D world, there are three axes—vertical, horizontal, and depth. In movement theory, these planes of motion are called frontal, sagittal, and traverse. So, when aligning the body, we don't *only* consider the ground up. We must also consider front to back and side to side. You want to create a 3D map of where each joint should be for a given posture.

Moving with the Breath, Expand and Contract

In yoga, most people know that we move. What is less visible is just how integral the breath is to this process. When we move, we move with the breath, propelled like a sale-ship at sea. The breath naturally creates movement in the body. Inhaling extends the spine and expands the body, while exhaling flexes the spine and compresses the body. For this reason, we inhale when entering a backbend and exhale when exiting a backbend. Conversely, we exhale when entering a forward bend and inhale when exiting the forward bend. When you do this consistently every time, you are well on your way to moving and breathing in the way that yoga intends.

"Moving with the breath, expanding and contracting" is not only limited to the spine during backbends and forward bends. This is where the real power of breath comes in. We can apply this principle of "inhale and expand", then "exhale and contract" to any muscle in a given posture. When you are in the posture, simply start by placing your attention on the desired muscle. On the inhale, activate the muscle you are focusing on. On the exhale, release and sink dipper, causing that muscle to relax and lengthen. You may further assist this lengthening by contracting an opposing muscle during your exhale. For example, say you want to lengthen the hamstring. On the inhale, you activate the hamstring, causing it to shorten. Then, on the exhale, you release and fold forward as the hamstring lengthens. During the exhale, you can use opposing muscles like the quads, abs, and even your arms to pull yourself further forward and lengthen the hamstring. No matter what muscle you use, each inhale and exhale is an opportunity to perform micro-movements, helping you go deeper into the posture

Ground and Rebound Effect

Ground and rebound is most easily seen in Tadasana, mountain pose. In this posture, we simply stand upright with our hands by our side. The ground and rebound effect occurs when we press our feet into the ground, causing our head to rebound up toward the ceiling. When you "ground" a certain body part by pushing it into a hard surface (like the ground or another part of the body), it tends to create a rebound effect, which causes another part of the body to move in the opposite direction. For every action, there is an equal and opposite reaction. The simplest example is tadasana, but you can do this in many different positions. For example, in plank pose (the top of a push up), you can press your hands toward the mat, causing the shoulders to round forward and the upper thoracic spine to "rebound" toward the ceiling. It is often favourable to press against your foundation as a means of extending and lengthening your body to the sky. Like the rapper, Mikeon, once said, "Touch the earth, puff the herb, then take flight like a Thunderbird." Same story here, but with less puffing of the herb.

Spirals

Western anatomy and physiology tend to view the body as a system of fulcrums and pullies, which move the body at right angles against the force of gravity. Yogis tend to view the body as a series of interconnected spirals. Dancers and martial artists often share this view.

To understand the concept of spirals, it is helpful to understand kinetic chains. This is the notion that joints and body parts affect one another during movement. When one joint is in motion, it creates a chain of events that put other joints into motion. These kinetic chains can move up the whole body from head to toe.

They resemble spirals because they invoke rotation around the body's centre axis. Visualise a martial artist doing a punch or roundhouse kick. It involves rotation of the feet, hips, trunk, and shoulders. But these spiralling rotations can exist all throughout the body on different scales, from subtle to gross. For example, in downward-facing dog, you want to rotate your wrists externally, which causes the biceps and shoulders to rotate outwards, and then the upper spine sinks deeper toward the mat. You can see how a subtle rotation can ricochet through the body. Viewing the body as a system of interconnected spirals rather than purely right angles can allow you much more dynamic and refined movement. It is about moving in curves, not just right angles. Even ask Shakira.

Psychedelic Techniques

The Elements

Each yogic posture and sequence can embody the elements. The elements are like a colour palette that fill the sketch of your asana. Below is a brief description of each element and its qualities within human movement.

Fire: Effort, power, strength, athleticism, tension, ambition, confidence, masculine.

Water: Free-flowing, effortless, fluid, supple, easeful, graceful, yielding, feminine.

Wind: Fast-moving, mobile, light, airy, weightless. That which moves things.

Earth: Structured, solid, stable. That which binds things.

Ether or Space: Emptiness. Pure Consciousness. The mental aspect. Real-time awareness of your body in space and time. Thought, intuition, guidance, refinement. Vision.

Masculine and Feminine

Each yoga pose is an expression of masculine and feminine forces coming into perfect balance.

Masculine is strong, rigid, tense, stable, moving at right angles.

Feminine is soft, supple, fluid, sensual, moving in rounded angles.

You may see some parallels with the elements here.

You can also think of masculine as a pure vision of the body in space and time, while feminine is a pure feeling of the body in space and time.

Each posture will have masculine and feminine forces active within it. We require strength and stability to hold our body in each position. We also require suppleness and fluidity to refine our position and accentuate it with style.

Perfect Grooves

It may sound like a simple concept, yet it is a very profound experience. The perfect groove happens when you enter a posture and continue refining it, until you hit a certain "ping" like a musical note. It is like a key fitting into a latch, unlocking the perfect posture. In this position, every muscle that needs to be activated is fully activated. Every muscle that needs to be yielding and open is fully open. The body locks into place, creating a structure of perfectly aligned balance from head to toe. In this mystical state of perfect alignment, a strong gust of vital energy flows through all the meridians, supporting the muscular-skeletal system as it floats effortlessly in space and time.

I wish to underscore the effortlessness. Half of your muscles feel dense and vital as they pull toward the ground, while the other half shoot up to the sky in their weightlessness. Half of your muscles are moving up, half of your muscles are moving down, while YOU stand stable at the nexus point of opposing forces.

These grooves feel timeless. There is the sense that what you are doing has been done by many great yogis before you. In that perfect posture, energy flow, and meditative alertness, you dissolve your personal ego and embody the spirit of yoga. Each posture is like an expression of an ancient archetype—that of the yogi. There is a timeless perfection therein.

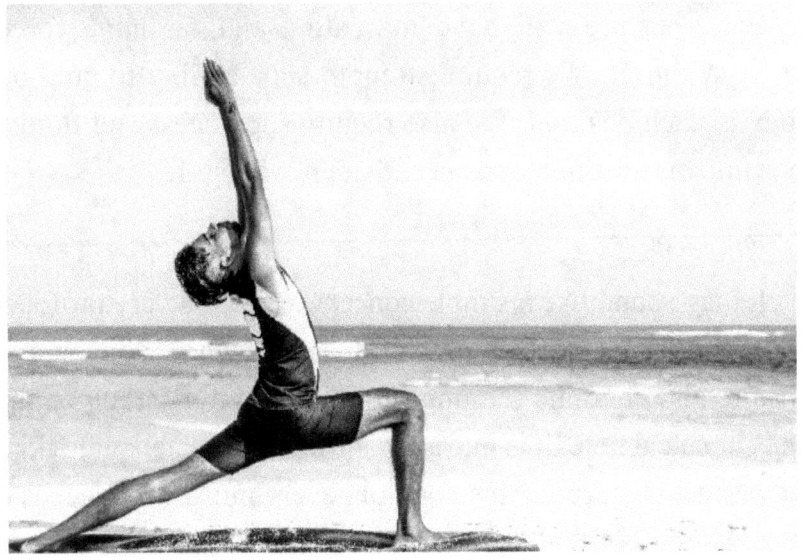

CHAPTER 3 – PRANAYAMA

"**P**ranayama is usually considered to be the practice of controlled inhalation and exhalation combined with retention. However, technically speaking, it is only retention. Inhalation/exhalation are methods of inducing retention. Retention is most important because it allows a longer period for assimilation of prana, just as it allows more time for the exchange of gases in the cells, i.e., oxygen and carbon dioxide."

"As long as the vayu (air) remains in the body, that is called life. Death is when it leaves the body. Therefore, retain vayu."

-Swami Muktabodhananda, The Hatha Yoga Pradipika

The Problem with Most Breathwork Sessions in Australia

I have attended several breathwork sessions in the last year and have seen some pros and cons.

On the positive side, they are well decorated with beautifully adorned rooms, epic soundtracks, and lots of people who add to the collective energy. All of this contributes to a juicy experience.

Yet what I would change in my own sessions is the programming of the breathing exercises. There is a common trend I have witnessed in each breathwork session. There is but one exercise, where people lay down and breathe at a fast tempo, in and out, for one hour straight.

In my view, this is no way to explore the wide and wonderful world of pranayama. There are many qualities of breath that go undiscovered when this is all that is done.

For one, it doesn't address breath retention. I believe that any bout of fast breathing should be followed by breath-holding. This is because they have opposing complementary effects. Fast breathing, also known as hyperventilation, increases our adrenalin, arousal, and oxygen to carbon dioxide ratio. On the other hand, breath-holding (hypoventilation) decreases our adrenalin, increases our carbon dioxide levels, and makes us feel very relaxed. To oscillate between the two is a form of contrast therapy. Most of us think of contrast therapy as jumping in and out of hot and cold water. This style of breathing works on a similar basis. We swing back and forth between two extremes, increasing our body's adaptive capacity.

It is essential to have the right balance of O_2 (oxygen) and CO_2 (carbon dioxide). CO_2 performs many vital functions in the body. It controls whether or not O_2 is released into the tissues, known as the Bohr effect. It dilates smooth muscles, such as the arteries, airways, intestines, and reproductive organs. It creates carbonic acid, which acts as a natural anti-oxidant and anti-histamine, thus lowering inflammatory markers. [Patrick McKeown 2015, Shut Your Mouth, Buteyko Clinic International]

Increasing our respiratory rate does not increase O2 levels, but it does decrease CO2 levels. This is because we tend to exhale more than we inhale. Plus, the process of delivering oxygen from the lungs to the cells via the arteries is a separate process to inhalation. Inhaling more O2 does not help this process. Yet lowering our CO2 levels with fast breathing will hinder this process.

Breathe more, and the more you need to breathe. Breathe less, and the less you need to breathe. Simon Borg-Oliver once said that we are fit based on how little we breathe, not how much. Picture an overweight person walking a small set of stairs, followed by them panting. On the other hand, a really fit person can take a short sprint and keep their breathing rate relatively the same.

Consider these words from Swami Muktabodhananda in the Hatha Yoga Pradipika:

"Pranayama is usually considered to be the practice of controlled inhalation and exhalation combined with retention. However, technically speaking, it is only retention. Inhalation/ exhalation are methods of inducing retention. Retention is most important because it allows a longer period for assimilation of prana, just as it allows more time for the exchange of gases in the cells, i.e., oxygen and carbon dioxide."

"When Prana moves, chitta (mental chatter) moves. When prana is without movement, chitta is without movement. By this steadiness of prana, the yogi attains steadiness and should thus restrain the vayu (air)."

"As long as the vayu remains in the body, that is called life.

Death is when it leaves the body. Therefore, retain vayu."

So, yes, retention is important. Yet there are many other qualities of pranayama to explore. You can adjust the ratio of inhale, exhale, internal retention, and external retention. This gives a sense of rhythm and tempo. You can focus on where the breath goes—lower abdomen, upper abdomen, intercostal (rib cage), and chest. You can even adjust which cavity the breath moves through, whether mouth, nose, or one nostril at a time. And how about bodily movements that accompany the breath? For instance, Bandhas or body locks, where you tense areas such as the anus, abdomen, and neck as a means of retaining the prana. When you explore the many different qualities of breath, you flex all your breathing muscles and entrain yourself for better respiration throughout daily life.

When it comes to the breathwork sessions I have attended recently, there is a value. These highly stimulating group experiences can be transformative. We get into a heightened state and process information that is different to the everyday. What I'm saying is that these shamanic sessions and the skill of breathing are two different things.

Breathe well, folks. Namaste.

Pranayama Exercises

Here is a set of pranayama practices, which I believe to be very well rounded. These exercises can energise you, relax you, and help you heal by removing tension. Best of all, they can be done in just a few minutes! Talk about high leverage.

Sama Vritti Pranayama – Box Breathing

Also called the fluctuating breath, "fluctuation" refers to the rhythm of the breath. The breath has four components—inhalation, internal retention, exhalation, external retention. To be clear, internal retention refers to holding the inhale in. External retention refers to holding the exhale out.

Box breathing refers to a specific ratio of these four components: 1, 1, 1, 1. For example, if you inhale for five seconds, you would hold at the top for five seconds, exhale for five seconds, then hold at the bottom for five seconds. This popular technique gets used in all sorts of special settings, from free-diving to the military. This is because a controlled ratio of breathing is a key which unlocks deep relaxation and focus.

While box breathing is a ratio of 1, 1, 1, 1, the fluctuating breath allows you to adjust the ratio. Generally, we would adjust the exhale to be longer. When your exhale and/or external retention is longer than the inhale, this activates the parasympathetic nervous system, i.e. relaxation response. Applying this can give us a ratio of 1, 1, 2, 1, or 1, 1, 2, 2. This is a perfect tool for relaxing the nervous system.

Creating a Full Breath

There is one more important key that goes along with box breathing—creating a full breath. This is achieved by consciously filling the three main cavities of the breath—the abdomen, the intercostal, and the chest. You will know the diaphragm has been engaged when the inhale causes your abdomen to expand and poke out. The intercostal is engaged when your rib cage and lats expand out to the side. And finally, the chest will expand by broadening at the front. When you exhale, you can notice each of those areas compress and get smaller again. During box breathing, you want all three of those areas to expand then contract with each breath.

Kapalbhati – Breath of Fire

Kapalbhati is an exercise where you breathe in and out through the nostrils at a fast tempo. This style of fast-paced breathwork energises and stimulates the nervous system.

Start by filling your lungs with a full breath. Tense the abdomen to sharply exhale 50% or less of the air from your lungs, causing your belly to move toward the spine. Then instantly "rebound" into an inhale, so the belly sticks out again. Let the exhale and inhale bounce like a basketball, with a tempo of about one breath cycle per second. You don't need to exhale and inhale your entire breath each time. We are only playing with the "top" 50% of your air, while the bottom 50% stays in you. Do roughly 20 of these fast breaths, followed by a complete exhale. Then do either a breath-hold with empty lungs, or take a full inhale and hold with full lungs. Hold for between 20 seconds and two minutes. Repeat for two or three rounds. As mentioned earlier, the benefit of breath-holding is greater assimilation of prana and greater relaxation.

Alternative option: You can try this technique with inhaling or exhaling through the mouth as well as the nose.

Nadhi Shodhan Pranayam: Alternate Nostril Breathing

In this pranayama, you breathe in and out through alternating nostrils. This has the effect of balancing and cleansing our nadis (subtle-energy channels) because the right and left nostrils are connected with the ida and pingala nadis respectively. These two are connected with The Sushamna nadi, which make up three major nadis in the body.

The sushamna nadi runs straight up the spine. The ida nadi and pingala nadi also move up the base of the spine, but in a weaving snake-like motion as seen in the image below:

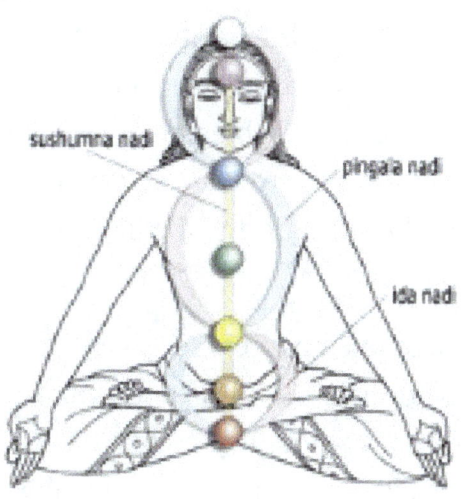

The ida nadi is yang or masculine. Its function is sun-like, promoting heat, physical energy, and activity. It connects to the right nostril. When we breathe in through the right nostril only, it stimulates and cleanses the ida nadi. The pingala nadi is feminine or yin. Its function is moon-like, promoting coolness, softness, relaxation, and reflection. The pingala nadi connects to the left nostril, so when we breathe in through the left nostril only, we stimulate and cleanse the pingala nadi.

In this exercise, we breathe in through the right nostril and then the left nostril in an alternating fashion, thus cleansing each major nadi and balancing our inner yin and yang forces. We do this by blocking off one nostril with our finger, so the air can enter or exit through only one nostril at a time. The breathing pattern resembles a pendulum, swinging from right to left. We breathe in through the right, then out through the left. Then in through the left, and out through the right. Repeat.

Regardless of whether you believe in the ida and pingala nadis, this exercise has some awesome benefits. Breathing through each individual nasal cavity helps to cleanse and open that cavity, thus creating a fuller breath. It also creates more strength and awareness in breathing muscles such as the diaphragm because it has to work harder to intaking oxygen through that small cavity. Lastly, the long and slow rhythm of this exercise has a very calming effect.

If you find that one nostril is relatively more blocked than the other, this is normal. The blocked nostril may even alternate at different times of the day/night. If your nostrils are particularly blocked, you can clear them with a netti pot. This apparatus allows you to pour salty water through one nostril and out of the other. It feels amazing. Just be sure to hold your breath while you pour—you don't want to accidentally inhale the water! There may be many fun substances to inhale through the nose, but water is not one of them.

CHAPTER 4 – MEDITATION

What is Meditation?

Everyone has at least a vague idea of what meditation is… the art of sitting on a cushion (or in a cave) repeating the word 'Om'. But let us go beyond stereotypes to look at a more essential definition of meditation.

In the yogic tradition, meditation (Dhyana) is the 7th limb of yoga and refers to "sustained focus". It is the practice of holding your attention on a single point for a prolonged period. The amount of time can vary from two minutes to sixty minutes. Furthermore, there are many options for where you can place your focus. It could be a candle flame, your breath, or a mantra you recite.

Yep, sustained focus on a single point. How simple and convenient. But I cannot help but be a rascal and throw a spanner in the works. In his lecture snippet, "Meditation is a very simple phenomenon", Osho says that meditation is not a state of doing…

"When you are doing nothing at all… physically, mentally, on any level at all… **that** is meditation. You cannot do it. You are only to understand it. Thinking is also doing. Concentration is also doing. Contemplation is also doing. When you are doing nothing at all, when you simply **are,** at your centre, utterly relaxed; That is meditation."

Naval Ravikant, a famous entrepreneur and philosopher, shared similar sentiments. He was asked, "So, what do you do? Do you focus on the breath, a mantra, what do you do?" Naval responded,

"Nothing, nothing, nothing… Because in meditation we are moving toward pure witnessing. Some of these practices help us get into that zone… but at the end what we are looking for is just pure witnessing".

In other words, meditation goes beyond the "act" of focusing. Focusing is a steppingstone. Our end game is tapping into pure witnessing, or pure observation.

Benefits of Meditation

States of Consciousness: From Doing to Being

This is where we enter the truth that happiness doesn't always come from material and external acquisitions. Whether you gain a woman, a house, or a piece of praise, the experience will only titillate you for so long. And then you are back in the throes of your own mind. Therefore, the most robust source of happiness is a peaceful state of mind.

What we learn through mediation is that we can feel amazing by simply doing nothing at all. Happiness is not a ledger of achievements. It is a state of consciousness. Its qualities include stillness, presence, engagement, fun, kindness, and humour. These are the tones of being we may often experience during or after meditation. Likewise, these are the tones we experience during any happy moment, whether hanging with friends, walking in nature, or sipping a morning coffee to the rising sun.

What these experiences all share in common is that we are submerged in the present moment, concerned less with the doing and more with the being. We drop the need to achieve anything in particular. We drop the need to manipulate, racing ahead to the next moment.

In meditation and in happiness, we arrive at THIS moment as the destination of contentment, the peaceful place where life can be enjoyed. It doesn't come from doing more and more… it comes from pausing and slowing down so we can savour this moment before it is gone. I believe the essence of higher consciousness is prioritising the being more than the doing.

Brain and Body: Western Concepts of Meditation

Relaxation

We have unpacked a major benefit of meditation—a serene state of consciousness, equipped to enjoy life. A sense of being more than doing. Yet there are extra embellishments we can add when thinking about the benefits of meditation.

Meditation shares a trait with pranayama, in that it brings us into the parasympathetic nervous system. It helps us to relax and unwind, to be at ease. This helps us with digestion, detoxification, and recovery.

Brain and Heart Coherence

Another benefit of meditation is improved brain and heart coherence. This concept refers to the level of communication and synchrony between all the brain regions, organs, hormones, and regulatory systems. Coherence and incoherence can be objectively monitored by observing brain scans and heart rate.

"Heart rate variability" monitors can reveal our coherence at a given time by measuring the tempo of our heartbeat. But different to a simple heart rate per minute, it measures the variability of our heart rhythm. A coherent state manifests as a sporadic heart rhythm, whereas a less coherent state manifests as a consistent rhythm. This may seem counter-intuitive. What happens is that our stress response creates a consistent and often faster heartbeat. Such is the vigilance of fight or flight. Whereas a relaxed heart can bump around at its own pace and leisure.

Coming back to the main point, meditation brings a sense of coherence to the body, heart, and brain, which can be scientifically observed. The result is greater communication between the whole brain and body, thus increasing our regulatory capacity.

The Default Mode Network: Becoming a Child Again

Another strong benefit of meditation is how it affects the default mode network. The default mode network (DMN) is the rut our brains get into. It's the groove of our neural networks, which dictate how we operate daily. It includes our habitual thoughts, judgements, emotions, and behaviours. Both meditation and psychedelics have the effect of disarming our default mode network. They weaken the habitual grooves and ruts that comprise our adult brain. We tap into a freshness, a wonder, a new way of doing things.

We still retain our knowledge and skill. And in fact, it gives us a performance advantage. When the DMN is dimmed, every neurone has the opportunity to communicate with other neurones it did not previously. Many possibilities open as the brain explores more of its own untapped potential. Novel connections, insights, and ways of doing and being can be accessed through meditation and psychedelics. These two practices move in the same direction—the expansion of one's mind.

Meditation Techniques

Now that we understand the benefits of meditation, let us explore some techniques. The aim of these practices is to cultivate a steady and sustained focus. From there, we may enter a meditative zone, where we drop the "doing" and access a deeper state of "being". The ultimate goal is to access pure witnessing and observation—the foundation of learning and insight.

Breathing Meditation

In this meditation, we focus on the breath. You may wonder how this is different from pranayama. Pranayama is more about the "doing" of breathwork. You try to execute various breathing techniques to achieve specific outcomes relating to the quality of your breath and body. With breathing meditation, it is less about executing the breath and more about observing the breath from a place of stillness. As mentioned, meditation is less about the doing and more about the being, the pure witnessing.

Chakra Meditation

While we have not dived deeply into the chakras, I feel compelled to share it here. I love this meditative technique—it is the bread and butter of my own practice. The chakras are seven energy centres running up the spine (or sushumna nadi). They are spiralling whirlpools of prana, which interface with different organs, bodily functions, and mental/emotional states. When every chakra is working well, you are at your peak of physical and spiritual health.

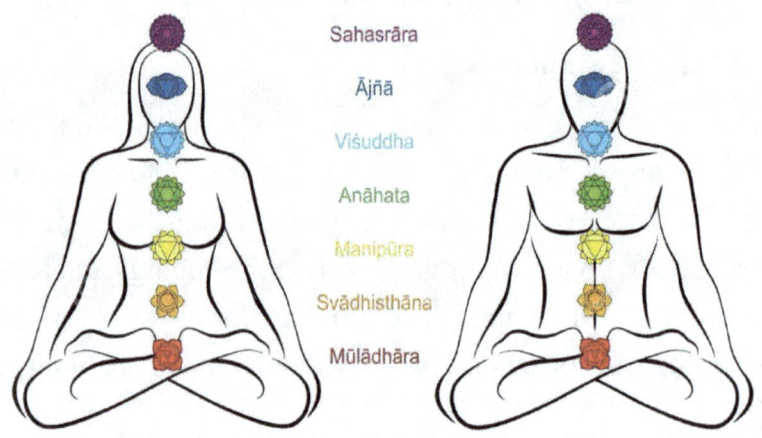

Sahasrāra

Ājñā

Viśuddha

Anāhata

Manipūra

Svādhisthāna

Mūlādhāra

A chakra meditation is when you engage with each chakra in any number of ways. You can breathe into them, vocalise, visualise, or recite affirmations which relate to that chakra. Whichever you choose, it is good to progress through each chakra from bottom to top.

Root chakra (Muladhara)
Location: Base of spine
Colour: Red
Affirmation: I am grounded, safe, secure, and comfortable.

Sacral chakra (Swadhisthana)
Location: Genitals
Colour: Orange
Affirmation: Vitality, vibrance, creative energy, and pleasure.

Solar plexus chakra (Manipura)
Location: Navel/abdomen
Colour: Yellow
Affirmation: Strength, power, potency. Capacity for action.

Heart chakra (Anahata)
Location: Heart
Colour: Green
Affirmation: Loving-kindness, appreciation, gratitude. Harmony, acceptance, and praise.

Throat chakra (Vishuddha)
Location: Throat
Colour: Blue
Affirmation: Communication and expression of divine truth. Creating with word as my bond.

Third eye chakra (Ajna)
Location: Between and behind the eyes
Colour: Purple
Affirmation: Vision, insight, intuition. Inner guidance and discernment.

Crown chakra (Sahasrara)

Location: Top of head and beyond

Colour: White light or Violet

Affirmation: Pure energy, pure consciousness, pure. inspiration. Enlightenment. Happiness, peace, love, Tao.

Visual Meditation

After doing some yoga/pranayama to elevate your energy, you may wish to gaze at a single point. You can choose either an external object or an internal object in your mind's eye. The former is easier when starting out, yet both have value. One great option is a candle flame. Flames are easy to stare at because they are mesmerising. Sinking into a visual point of focus is great for concentration and relaxation. Just be careful not to burn your finger or your house. You must sign a waiver at the end of this book.

Mantra Meditation

In this meditation, you recite a mantra. It can be English or Sanskrit, out loud or in your head. I would recommend trying some Sanskrit mantras out loud. They are very resonant and melodic, providing a pleasant medicine to the nervous system. Furthermore, Sanskrit mantras are said to be unique in that they contain the vibration of the concept they are describing. Hence when you recite the mantra, it has an extra pulling power for attracting that experience into your life. Here are some of my favourite Sanskrit mantras you may wish to try. Search them up to learn the melody.

Om Gum Shreem Maha, Lakshmiyei (luck-sh-meh-he-aye) Namaha: Universal power, remove all obstacles, to create an abundant increase of energy, so I may live my divine life-purpose to completion and praise.

Ong Namo, Guru Dev Namo: I bow to the creative power of the cosmos. I bow to the divine teacher within.

Om Tat Sat: The infinite spirit is the only truth.

Sat Nam: Truth is my name.

Om (Aum): The sound of the universal spirit. It is said to clear energy blockages.

Besides these Sanskrit mantras, you may wish to recite any English word or affirmation. Simply repeat the word/phrase, focusing deeper and deeper on its meaning. Words are spells. That's why we call it spelling.

Mindfulness Scanning Meditation

Instead of having one singular point of focus, this meditation allows you to shift your focus around like a torch. Slowly scan your body from head to toe, listen out for different sounds, or scan the visual environment. This exercise teaches us to observe and notice our environment—a rich tapestry that we often overlook.

Pure Consciousness or Stillness Meditation

Most of the meditations above have included an object as a point of focus. Whether it is a candle, a mantra, or the breath, these are all objects within the field of consciousness. In this meditation, we shift our awareness to the field of awareness itself. This can be quite a trippy meditation, fruitful for metaphysical insights. Whenever you notice your focus shift to an object, bring it back to the pure field in which the object exists. Bonus tip: It may be useful to do some pranayama and/or another meditation as a warm-up, and then drop into pure consciousness at the end.

CHAPTER 5 – THE YOGI'S GUIDE FOR LIFELONG PRACTICE

Consistency Each Day

Consistency for Health

It is a simple yet powerful teaching. Don't let simplicity fool you. I always tell my students, "It's better to do a few minutes every day than one hour once or twice per week." This is especially true for those in physical pain. Consistent movement is medicine. Mobility is health. When you go multiple days without yoga or movement, the muscles tend to seize up and become weak. On the other hand, when you move a little each day, you grease the groove of the muscular-skeletal system.

Consistency for Skill

Beyond wellness, daily practice increases performance. This is indicated by science. In Daniel Coyle's book, "The Talent Code", he refers to a study where two control groups were learning to play the piano for the first time. One group practiced for 10 minutes per day. The other group practiced twice per week for one hour each session. When the groups were assessed on their ability to play a song, the results were surprising: The first group performed much better.

This may be surprising because the second group had a larger sum of practice—120 minutes per week compared to 70 minutes per week. The researchers' interpretation is based on how the brain acquires and retains skill.

When we practice a skill, we begin carving the relevant neural networks. Thousands of neurones must switch on and communicate with painstaking precision. The more consistently we practice a skill, the more we "grease the groove" of those neural networks, strengthening and refining their pathways. In his book, Coyle refers to myelin, a fatty substance in the brain that acts as insulation and lubricant for our synaptic pathways. When we practice a skill on a given day, our brain will insulate that pathway with myelin, thus increasing the speed and accuracy of the electrical signals. When we go a week without practicing the skill, our myelin pathways can weaken, and we have to play catch-up to cover lost ground. Therefore, daily practice for just 10 minutes will help to sustain those greasy neural networks, thus helping you to maintain and develop your skill.

Follow-Along Video Flows

If you're a beginner who is yet to learn and master a yogic sequence, obviously you need an instructor to guide you through it. If attending classes every day is not an option for you, perhaps videos on YouTube or an app is ideal. The benefit of this is flexibility. Each morning, lunch, and evening, you can search up a yoga flow of your desired length, difficulty, and theme. For example, you may search: "10-minute morning yoga for beginners." Given the size of the world wide web, I'm sure you could find a yoga flow for just about anything. Just don't get too kinky. Using online videos will enable you to practice yoga in your own location, on your own schedule, whether you're a complete newbie or advanced sage. Technology can be a great tool when used in moderation for the right reasons.

Classes Each Week

While it's great to practice on your own, there is an extra benefit in attending group classes each week. You will gain a sense of community, meeting like-minded people on a similar path. You will also gain access to an experienced teacher. They can provide you with new flows, postures, and specific feedback on a technique. Plus, great teachers will remind you about the big picture of yoga and what we are trying to achieve on and off the mat.

Independent Practice, Especially Outdoors

So far, we have spoken about "follow along" types of yoga, whether it was following a video or a live teacher in the classroom. The next essential step is walking outside and leading yourself through a practice. This is an opportunity to internalise the rhyme, reason, and structure of a yoga flow, while adding your own unique flavour. You will gain some awesome benefits from your independent yoga. For one, you can focus solely on yourself rather than a leader, freeing up more presence for your own body and breath. Another benefit is pure independence. You can fit in a yoga session anywhere, anytime, with no resource other than yourself. I also recommend doing these solo sessions outdoors every so often, if not daily. You will feel a greater surge of vital energy when you are outside among the elements. You will become one of the trees blowing in the wind.

Always do Pranayama and Meditation, At Least for Several Minutes

It is much easier to stay consistent with your asanas, pranayama, and meditation when you stack them all together. It is easier to schedule. But more importantly, these three practices meld and synergise nicely together, creating a well-rounded spiritual practice. Asanas boost our circulation and move energy through the body. Then, taking a seat for pranayama, we use the breath to further refine this flow of vital energy. Meditation is the finish line, where we take our hand off the wheel and witness the brilliance of what we have created. Well, it's what God has created, we just wiped the stains from our windshield.

Small Yoga Snacks vs Long Yoga Sessions

A yoga session can honestly be very short yet highly beneficial. Likewise, it can also be long and highly beneficial. Size doesn't matter—it's how you use it. When you are aware of these possibilities, you can choose different lengths of yoga sessions for different times of the day or week. For example, look at my own routine. I do a sun salutation sequence every morning, and a moon salutation sequence every evening before dinner. Each one takes 20 or 30 minutes, including sitting and breathing at the end. These are my non-negotiables. Every day I get in these two short yoga flows. Some days, I add a longer session in the middle of the day, or do a more intense workout with yoga as a cool down.

Once you start implementing self-led yoga flows, you can take many yoga snacks or meals throughout the day at your own convenience. The minimum I recommend is once per day, and up to three or four per day is very doable. The analogy of "snacks and meals" is appropriate here because yoga sessions are a form of nourishment. It will genuinely increase your energy levels, motivation, and sense of peace… perhaps even more than eating food. If you do a little less eating and a little more yoga, you will be surprised by the results. Bon Appetit.

Private Lessons

In the last couple of passages, we spoke about independence. Now the pendulum swings the other way toward the benefit of mentorship. As with most skill-sets, finding an instructor to take you through private lessons is essential to reaching the highest level. A personal instructor can give you 100% attention and tailored feedback. Plus you don't need to do private lessons all the time—you can do them every now and then as it takes time to implement the pointers. One last tip is to know your intended focus when you go to your instructor, so they can help you address your greatest curiosity or obstacle.

Research Alignment Cues

The pendulum now swings back to independence. There are many rocks to pick up and look underneath along your yogic journey—community classes, YouTube classes, private lessons and personal practice. The next rock is your self-led effort to learn some theory. It can be invaluable to read or watch instructional content that teaches you the alignment cues of a specific posture. It is very common for the aspirant (including myself) to practice a posture over and over until, one fateful day, you learn a new adjustment which transforms the posture completely. It is like escaping the matrix.

But please don't rush this process unnecessarily. Don't get drowned in theory, micro-managing, and analysing every point of your body all the time. You must find the balance of masculine and feminine, logic and feeling. Remember to enjoy your flows and savour the moment. Feel pleasure and gratitude for your body, breath, and Qi. But each week or month, learn how to improve a posture of choice by reading an article about its finer details. YouTube can also be great for this. As the months and years roll over, you will be surprised by how many postures you know inside out. Eventually, the perfect posture becomes one with your intuitive expression.

Consider Doing a Teacher Training One Day

This may not be for everyone, but if you LOVE yoga, then I would highly recommend it. This section is a taste test of what YTT can do for you.

Reflecting on my own YTT, it is simultaneously the most challenging and rewarding thing I have ever done. The challenge came from the sheer volume and intensity of effort. They were very long days. For a month, we were studying and practicing over 12 hours per day for six days per week, from 6 am to 7.15 pm. The whole day was filled with asana practice, lectures, and meditation, plus meal breaks. In addition to this intensive schedule, we needed to work on assessment pieces like writing articles, studying for an exam, and creating our first yoga flow, which we would lead our fellow students through. If I had to sum it up in one word, it would be "intensive".

But while it was painful and difficult at times, it ended up being the best decision and investment I ever made. One of the most obvious benefits is that I walked away with a solid foundational blueprint of yoga. It really clarified my understanding of what yoga is, what the benefits are, and how to perform it well while teaching others. But the education you receive is far from complete. Rather, it is just the beginning. It piques many more questions, revealing more trails to explore. It is up to the aspirant to continue the journey. Still, the initial 200hr teacher training is the perfect foundation to build from.

Another huge benefit I received from YTT was the opportunity to start teaching. Educating and inspiring others, both locally and on the internet, has been a huge source of fulfilment in my life… not to mention a nice boost to my finances. Teaching has also helped me to meet people and make new friends. It is an enriching, pro-social experience. And it won't leave you washed up like a nightclub!

APPENDIX: ALIGNMENT CUES FOR POPULAR ASANAS

I could give pages of alignment cues for each given posture, but that would be cumbersome for us both. And so, I have provided a sketch, a starting point. It's up to you to fill in the gaps, to figure some things out for yourself. The joy is not in reading the most thorough analysis, but in using your own intelligence through the art of doing.

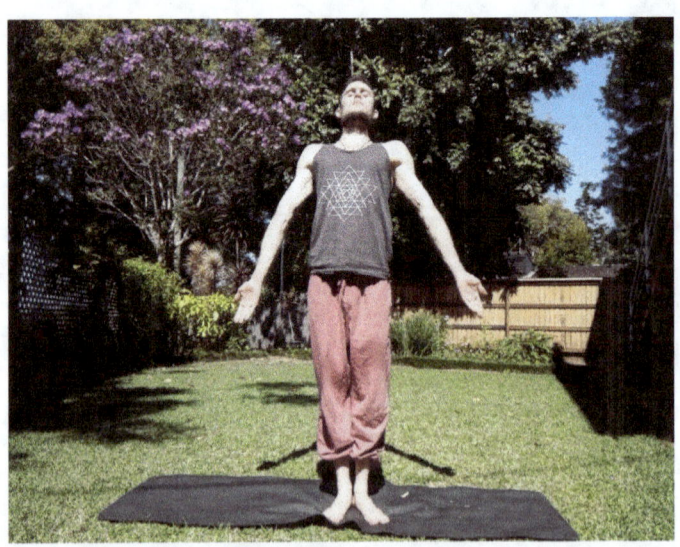

Mountain Pose (Tadasana) – Your feet are together, facing forward. Press the ball of your foot into the mat, lifting the arches. Externally rotate at the ankles, knees, and hips. Pelvis is neutral, like a bucket full of water that you cannot spill. Spine extends upward to the ceiling. Move shoulders up, back, then down. Externally rotate your arms at the shoulder joint so the arms are by your side with your palms facing forward. Neck is directly above spine, with crown floating upwards.

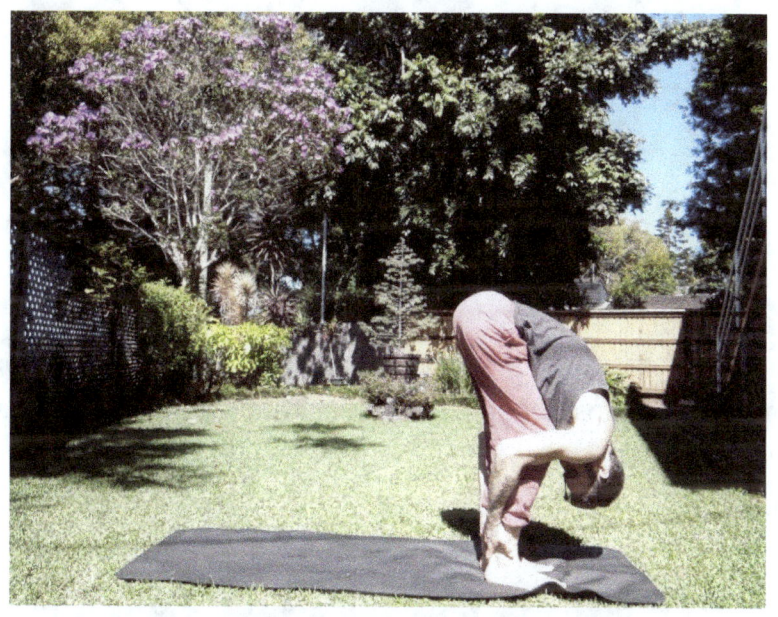

Standing Forward Fold (Uttanasana) – Entering from Tadasana, exhale and hinge at the hips, bending knees slightly as you fold forward while keeping the spine straight. At the bottom of the forward fold, bend your knees generously so that your abdomen is touching your thighs. For hand positioning, you may hold your elbows, grip your ankles, or "pistol grip" your big toes. It is safe to relax the shoulders and round the spine so long as your knees are bent. Caution: if you fold forward and the knees are straight, the spine should also be straight. If you round the spine with knees fully straight, it can place pressure on the lower back.

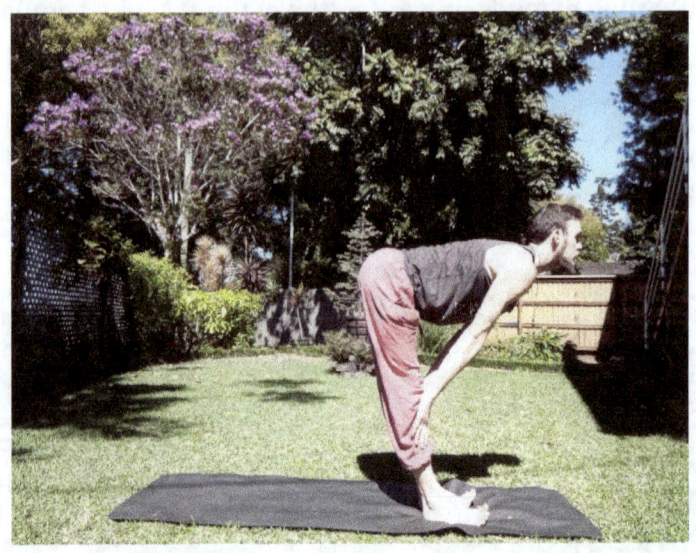

Halfway Lift (Ardha Uttanasana) – Entering from standing forward fold, inhale as you straighten your legs, hinge up from the hips, lengthen the spine, drawing your shoulders down and back while tilting the neck up to look forward. You then exhale and re-enter the standing forward fold.

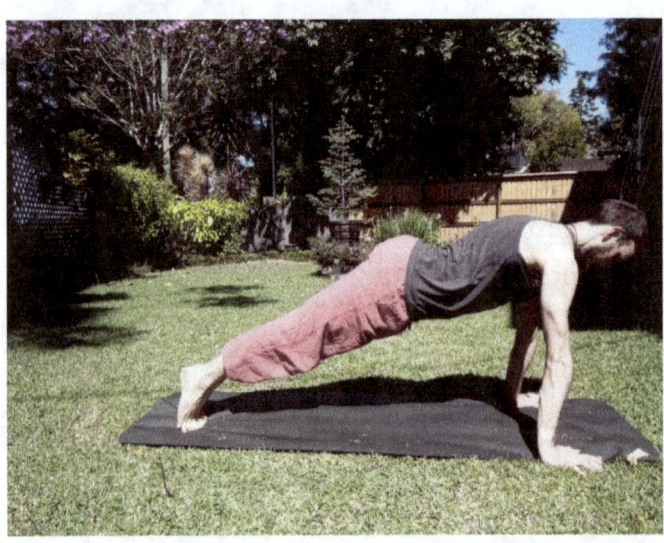

Plank (Phalakasana) – Entering from standing forward fold, place palms on front of the mat directly below each shoulder. Step each foot back toward the back of the mat. In plank, tuck the pelvis forward so the abdomen tightens. Inhale to extend the thoracic (upper) spine. Exhale and press into the ground with your palms so the shoulders round forward a little, yet not over-accentuating a rounded upper back.

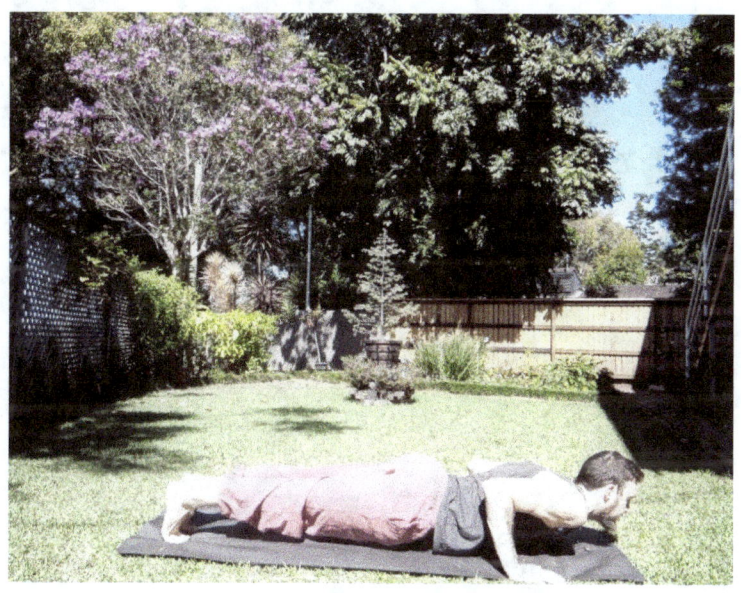

Four-Limbed Staff Pose (Chaturanga Dandasana) – Exhale from plank and bend at the elbow joint, lowering your whole body towards the mat. Keep the pelvis and abdomen tucked. Keep elbows close to the side of your body, not flailing out. Hold the position so your torso and hips are floating just above the ground. If this posture is too challenging, drop the knees to the mat first before lowering down (eight-limbed staff pose).

Eight-Limbed Staff Pose (Astangasana) – Similar to chaturanga but with the knees, chest, and chin on the mat for extra support. Chaturanga is called "four-limbed staff pose" because you have four "limbs" touching the mat—two palms and two feet. With the eight-limbed staff pose, the four additional limbs include your two knees and two pecs (chest muscles).

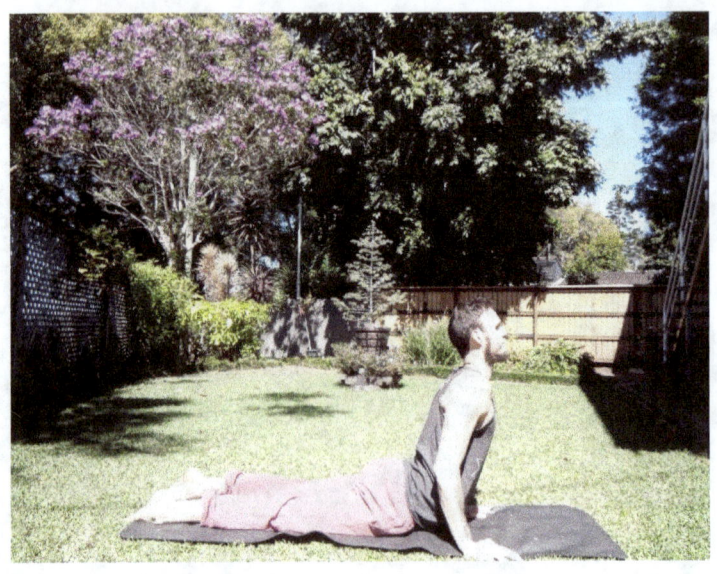

Cobra (Bhujangasana) – From the eight-limbed or four-limbed staff pose, push your hands into the mat and start straightening your arms to lift your chest. The chest is now facing the front of the room. Keep your arms slightly bent. The feet are in plantar flexion, meaning the toes are extended away from your head. Your legs, hips, and pelvis are all on the ground. On an inhale, extend and lengthen the thoracic spine, drawing the shoulders down and back. This is our first back-bending shape.

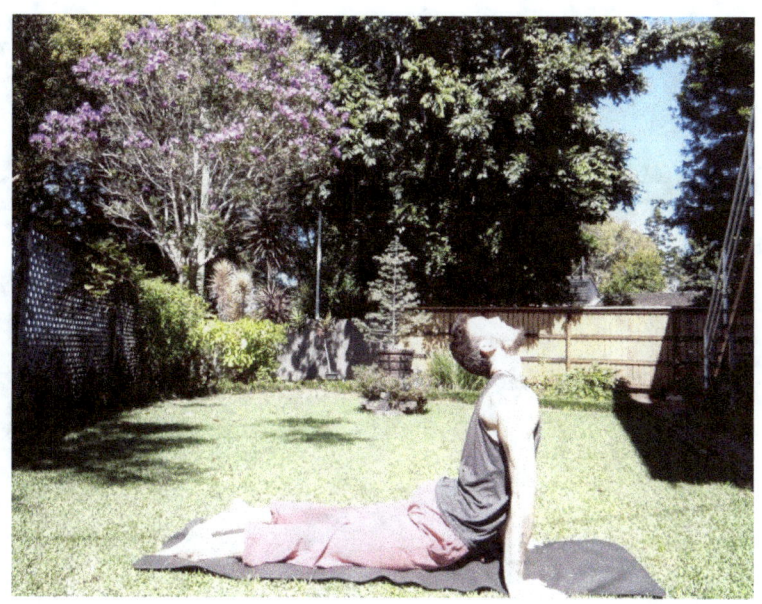

Upward **Facing Dog (Urdhva Mukha Svanasana)** – Entering from cobra or chaturanga, straighten your arms fully so the chest faces the front of the room and the head is tall toward the ceiling. The knees, hips, and pelvis hover above the mat, so only your feet and hands are supporting you. Contract your quads, hip flexors, and rear delts to "pull yourself forward", accentuating the back. Inhale to extend the thoracic spine, draw the shoulders down and back, and perhaps look to the ceiling.

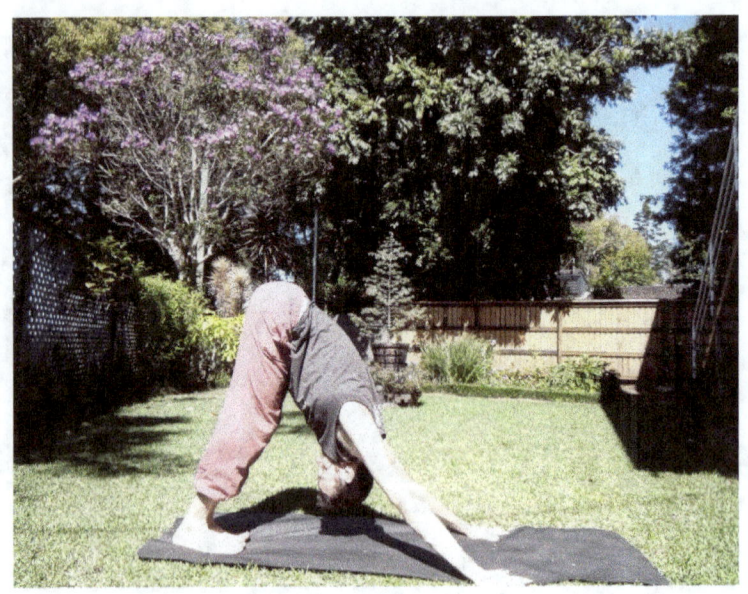

Downward-Facing Dog (Adho Mukha Svanasana) – From the upward facing dog, lift your pelvis off the mat and move toward plank. Then move your butt toward the ceiling, creating an upside down "V". From here, you can bend the knees as the focus is on creating a long and extended spine. Tilt the pelvis to neutral or slightly back (anterior tilt), letting the lower spine sink deeper toward the mat. Let the upper spine extend or arch slightly, scapular and shoulders broadening, and chest opening. With hands planted, subtly rotate shoulders externally, and forearms internally. Let the neck relax, with crown of the head sinking toward the mat.

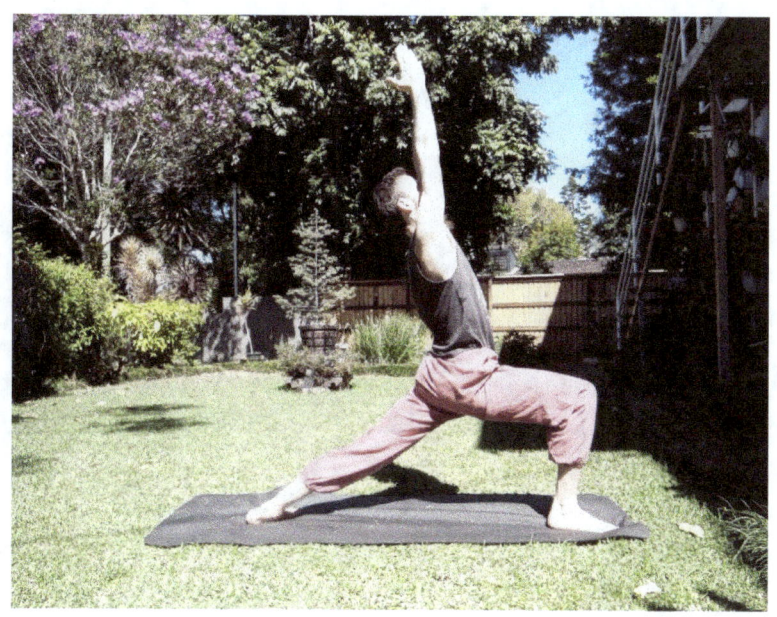

Warrior 1 (Virabhadrasana I) – Entering from downward dog, roll forward to plank and bring the right knee to chest, then place the right foot at the front of the mat with toes facing forward. Ground the left foot at a 45-degree angle, with both arch and heel on the mat. Inhale as you hinge up at the hips and lift arms overhead. Ensure the hips are neutral and square, so draw the left hip forward and the right hip back. Move energy upward through the lats and arms, then ground the shoulders down and back. To exit, bring arms down by the side, exhale as you hinge forward at the hips, place palms on the front of the mat, return to plank, then chaturanga, upward facing dog, downward-facing dog, then repeat on the other side (left foot forward).

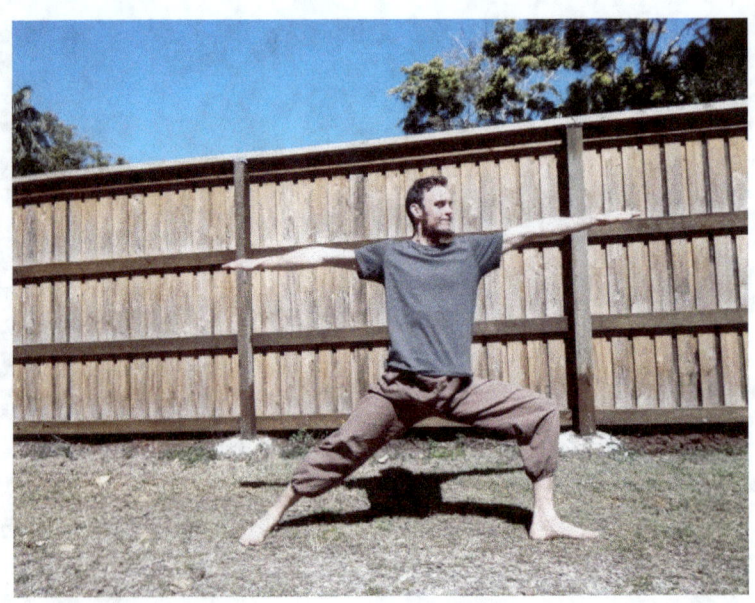

Warrior 2 (Virabhadrasana II) – Entering from Warrior 1, externally rotate your back (left leg) so that your toes and hips are now facing the side of the mat, while the right toes still face the front of the mat. Keep your right knee bent, positioned above your right ankle or slightly behind. Do not let your knee collapse inward—keep that leg externally rotated. Keep hips and torso facing the side of the mat. The arms come out by your side and turn your head to look to the front of the mat.

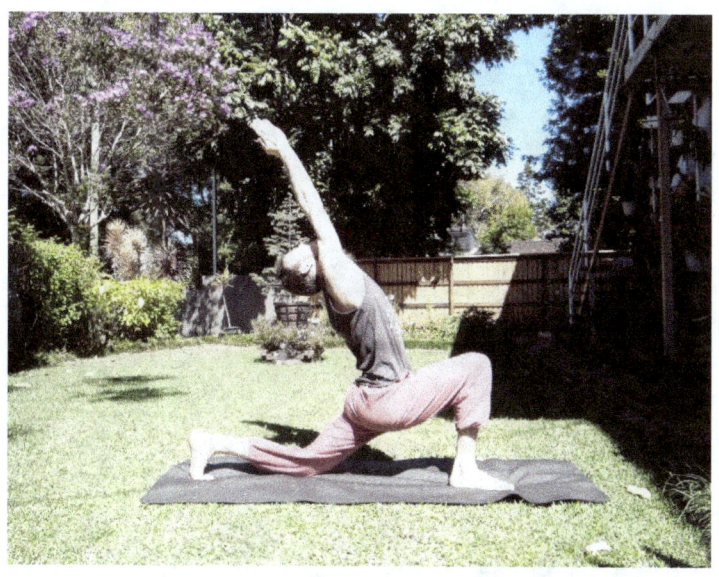

Low Lunge (Anjaneyasana) – Entering from the downward dog or plank, bring the right foot forward to the front of the mat. Bring the left knee to the ground. Inhale as you lift the palms to the sky. Exhale as your hips sink deeper into the ground, then shoulders draw down and back. To exit, inhale as you bring arms down by your side, place palms on the front of the mat, lift knee off the ground, either return the right foot back for plank or bring the left foot forward to front of mat, in standing forward fold.

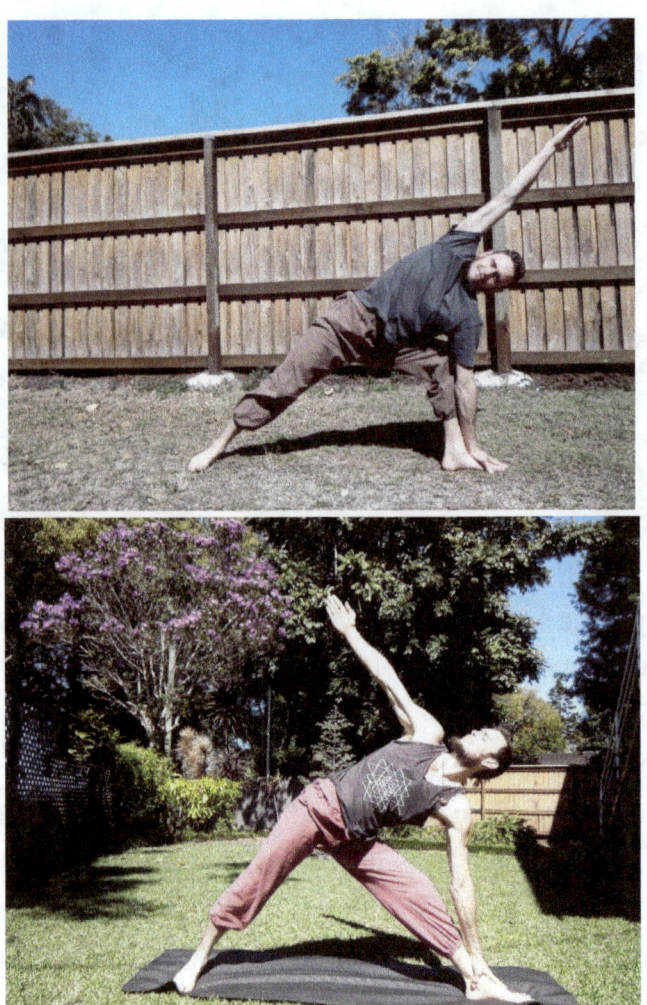

Standing Postures – Extended. This will include the alignment cues for *Extended Triangle (Utthita Trikonasana)* and *Extended Side Angle (Utthita Pasvakonasana)*, as these postures share a lot in common. The main difference is that, in triangle, you straighten the front leg before entering, whereas with side angle, the front leg is bent at the knee. In both cases, the hips and torso are facing the side of the mat. The back foot is also facing the side of the mat, and the front foot is facing the front of the mat. Extend the arms out by your sides. Move the right arm toward the front of the mat by folding at the spot where your right oblique connects with your right hip. Go as far as you feel comfortable, then place your right palm on your ankle, foot, or floor. With extended side angle, you can also place the right elbow on your right knee. In these postures, you want your front foot, front knee, two shoulders, and head all to be vertically stacked so you can fit between two narrow windowpanes.

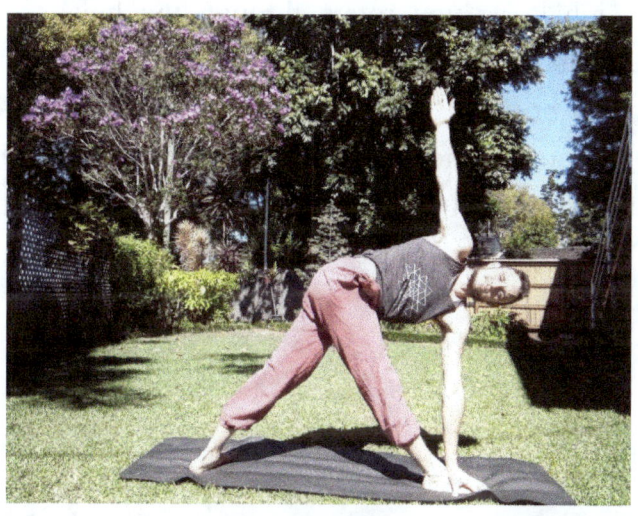

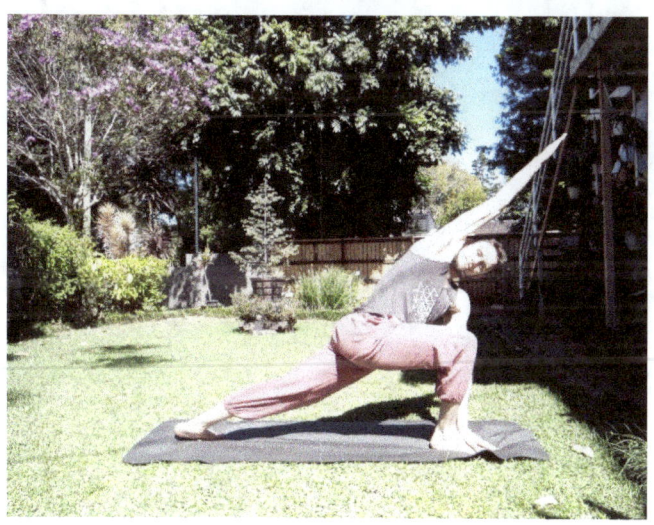

Standing Postures – Revolved. This includes *Revolved Triangle (Parivrtta Trikonasana)* and *Revolved Side Angle (Parivrtta Pasvakonasana)*. From Warrior 1 position, if you are going into revolved triangle, start by straightening your front leg. For revolved side angle, keep the front leg bent. Inhale and take your left arm in the air, and your right hand on your hip. Exhale as you hinge forward at the hips. Place your left palm on your right foot or on the mat. Keeping the left hand planted, inhale as you rotate through the hips, torso, and shoulders, taking the right arm to the sky. Try to extend your spine while bringing your torso closer to the inside of your right leg. More advanced versions of triangle and side angle do diverge, yet the most entry level versions are very similar.

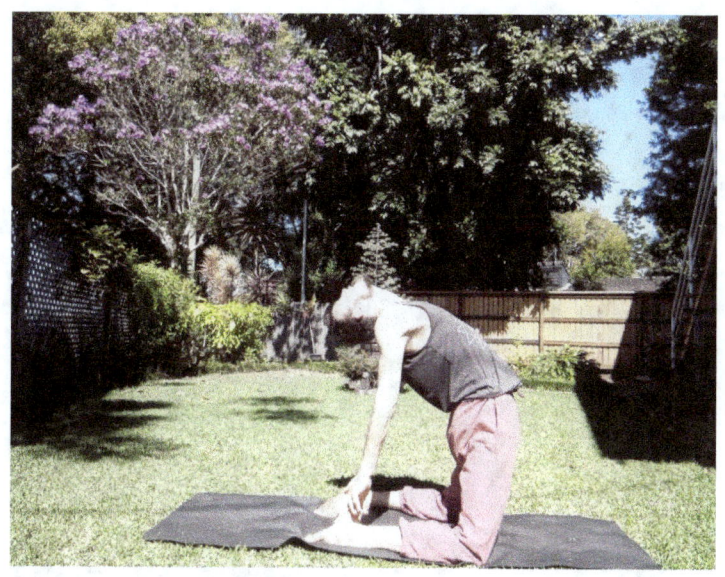

Backbends – This can include the postures *Camel (Ustrasana), Locust Pose (Salabhasana), Bow Pose (Dhanurasana), and Wheel (Urdhva Dhanurasana).* Different backbends have different cues, yet we will focus on the universal aspects. In all cases, we are wanting to extend the spine. This is the primary goal. Prioritise extending the spine, even if other parts of the movement are less accentuated. The glutes are an interesting one here. You may want to engage the glutes at first to push your hips forward. However, you may then want to relax your glutes because tense glutes can create a tense lower back, which limits the range of motion in the backbend. So, relax the glutes. Shoulders externally rotate, drawing them back and down (retraction and depression). The final step is to let the neck hang back, but only if it feels comfortable.

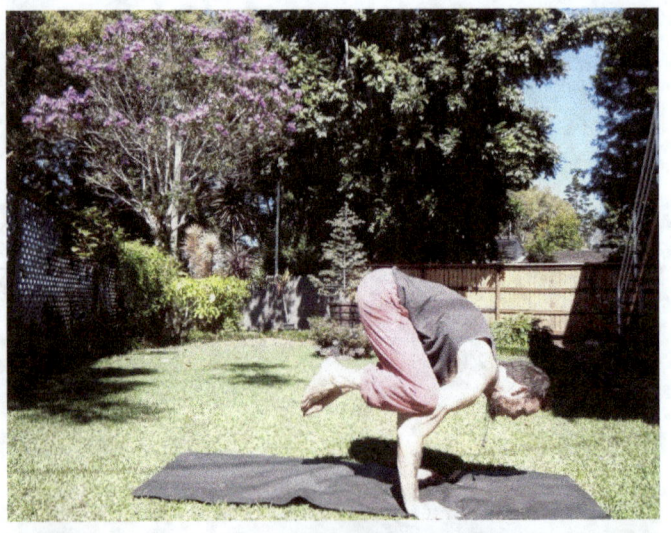

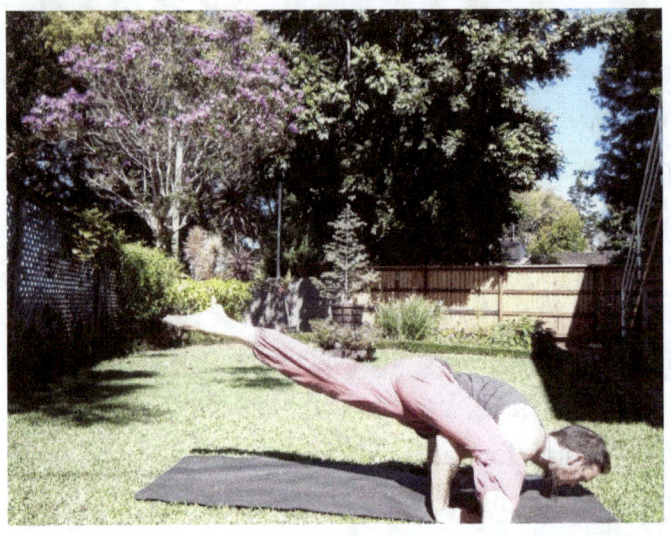

Arm Balances – This includes the arm balances that are not fully inverted. Let us include *Crow (Bakasana), Firefly Pose (Tittibhasana), and Eka Pada Koundinyasana*, plus more. The stability in these postures comes from strong engagement in the hands and wrists, triceps, shoulders, and core. Therefore, a large part of mastering these postures is learning to switch on and engage those muscles. Starting from the ground up, place your palms on the mat with hands thoroughly engaged and fingers spread quite wide. Press sternly into your foundation, which will activate the triceps and shoulders. Have arms tucked in close to the body. Perhaps one or both knees are supported by your triceps. Then lift your feet off the ground, engaging the core however much is necessary for that posture. Bonus tip: Be willing to fall forward. Only by going to each extreme will you truly find the balance point. I suggest landing on your crown or forehead, while also supporting yourself with your arms. If you fall on your nose, it will hurt. The crown won't hurt so much.

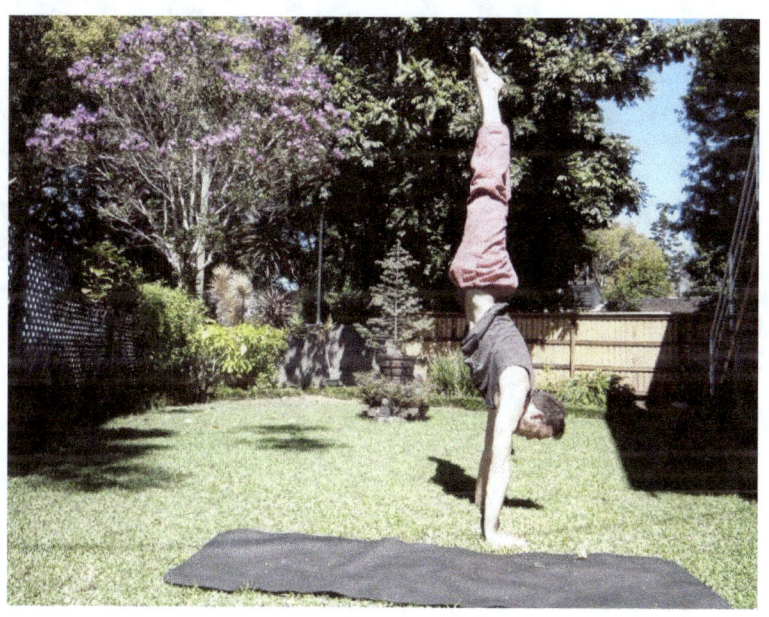

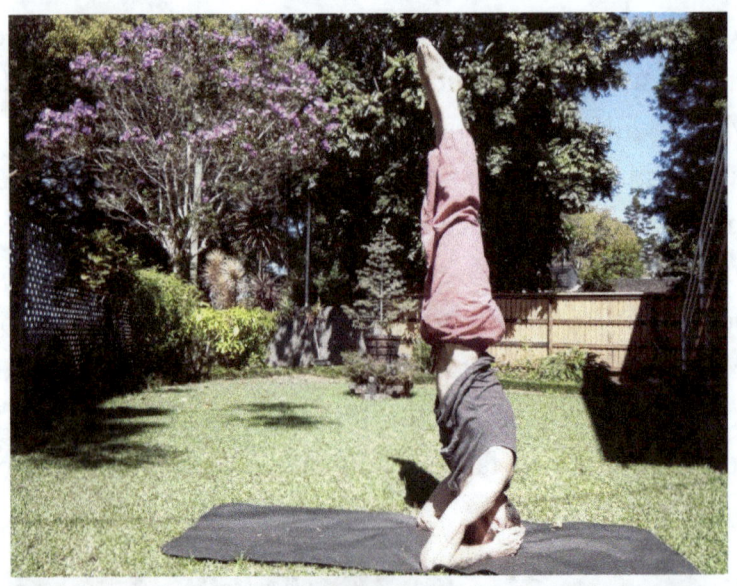

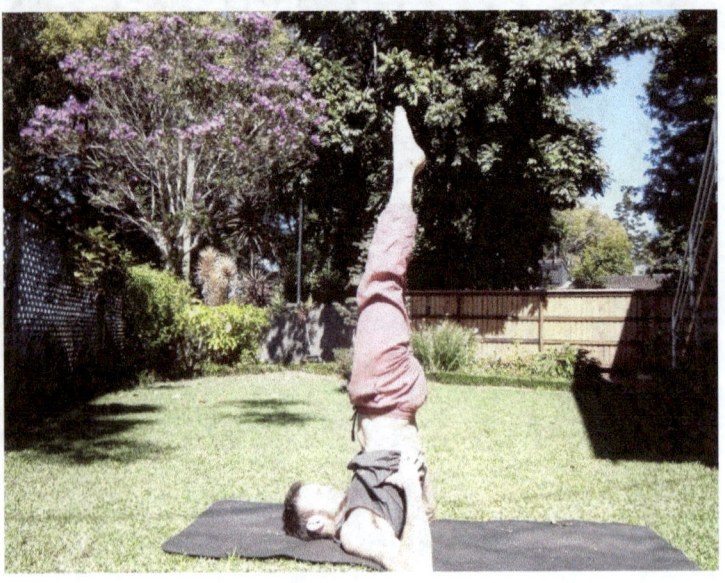

Inversions – This will include handstand (Adho Mukha Vrksasana), forearm stand (Pincha Mayurasana), headstand (Sirsasana), and shoulder stand (Sarvangasana). Inversions are about stacking over your centre of gravity by learning to engage the right muscles. The ones closest to your foundation (the floor) take the most precedence, and then as you move upward, the muscles become less pivotal. However, engaging every muscle can help you in the early stages. The ground and rebound effect is relevant here. You want to press against your foundation, whether it is with your hands, forearms, or elbows. This helps the rest of your body to extend vertically toward the sky. If you don't extend enough, your feet will fall back the way they came. If you over-extend, the feet will move past your head and fall on the other side. So, the key is in "catching" yourself mid-air. This catching comes from engaging certain muscles. From bottom to top, this would include using the hands, arms, shoulders, core, glutes, and perhaps even thighs. If you tense these muscles, they can help you secure your body. The more stable and strong the lower muscles are (in this case, the hands, forearms, and shoulders), the more wiggle room you have to let the upper muscles relax and float about.

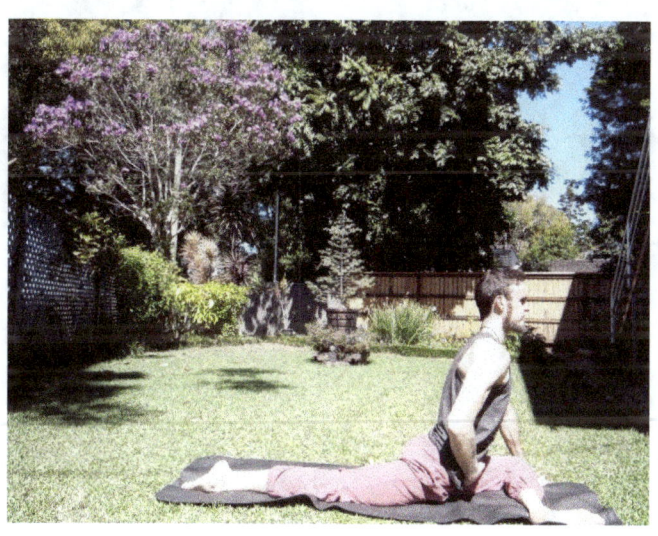

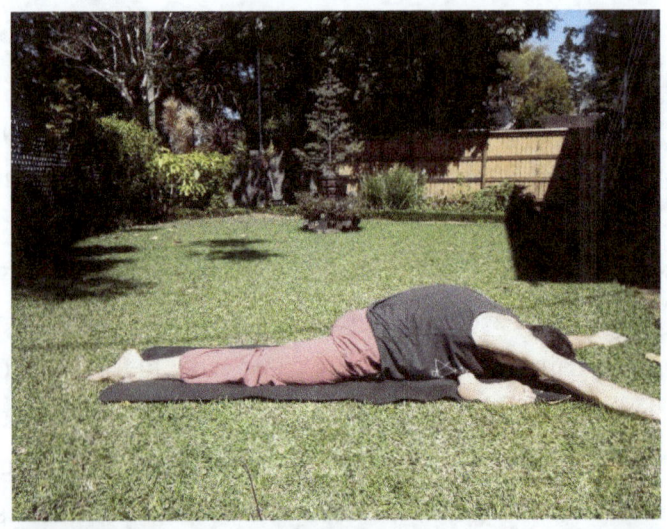

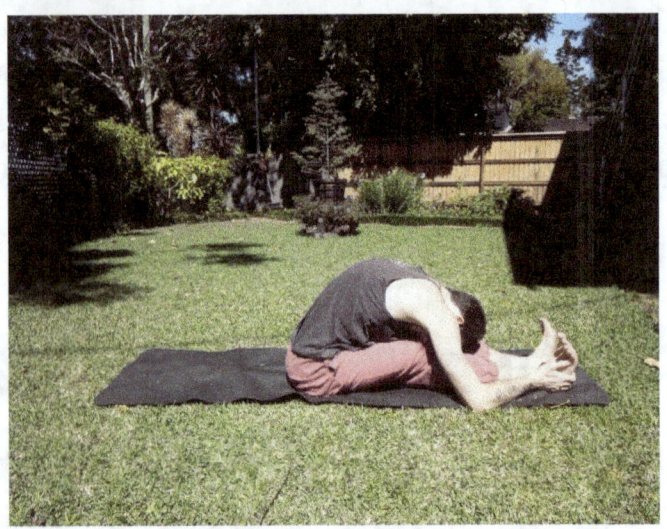

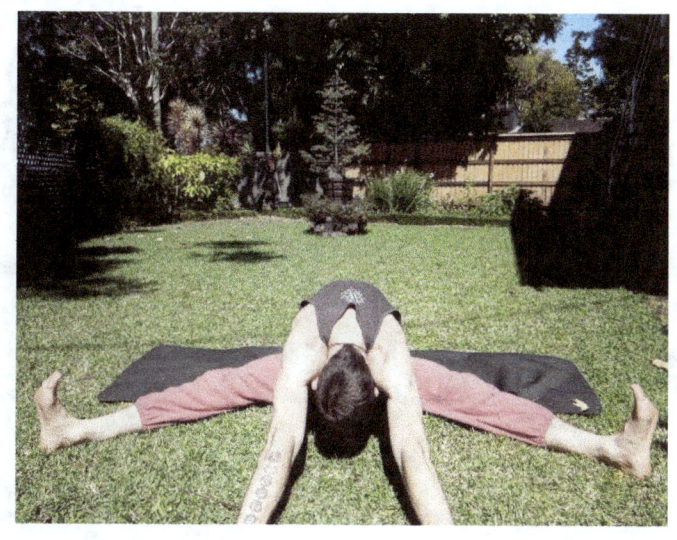

Forward Folds – This may include seated forward bend (Paschimottanasana), seated straddle forward fold (Upasvistha Konasana), or pigeon (Eka Pada Rajakapotasana). Sitting with your legs in position, inhale and extend the spine, creating a sense of space. Then exhale as you forward fold at the hips. A big part of forward folding is perseverance—with each breath, you move a little deeper into the posture. With each inhale, you extend the spine, coming up a little bit. Then exhale as you sink deeper through the hips, relaxing the spine. You are taking one step back and two steps forward, with each inhale and exhale. During straight-legged forward fold and straddle, it can be good to contract the quads on the inhale, creating the sense of pulling your legs back toward yourself. Then as you exhale, you contract the abdomen to help yourself hinge further forward. You can also use your hands to grip your feet like a handle, pulling yourself further forward.

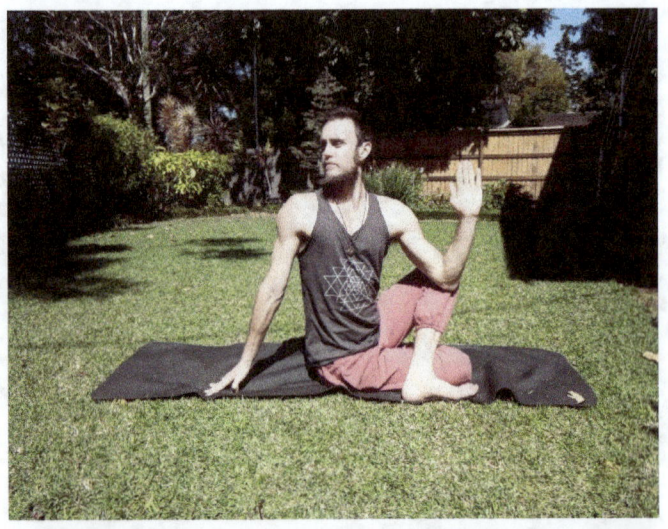

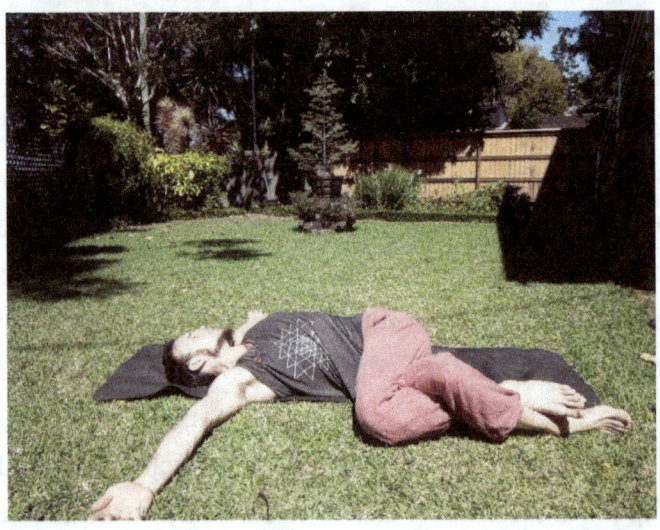

Twists – I like to do a reclined twist at the end (Supta Matsyendrasana), yet this could also include half lord of the fishes (Ardha Matsyendrāsana). Before entering a twist, we inhale to extend the spine and create space. Then exhale as we enter the twist. Starting from bottom to top, we rotate through the hips, spine, shoulders, and neck. When exiting, we do the reverse. Exhale as you exit with the neck, shoulders, spine, and hips.

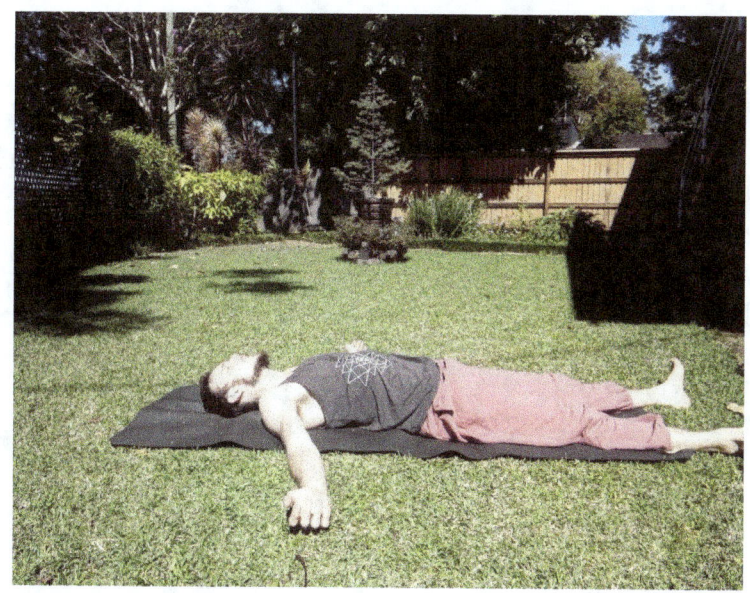

Shavasana (dead body/corpse pose)- This posture is performed at the end of your session. The intention is to become deeply restful, utterly relaxed, as your body absorbs the practice. You want your body to be symmetrical, with the arms and legs rotating slightly outwards. The pelvis is neutral, and the spine is long. Wiggle about until you enter this place. You may want to place something over your eyes, to darken the visual scene. Take a deep breath, and fall into oblivion.